FAT LOSS

WORKOUT PLAN

THE FLIGHT OF ICARUS

*SHRED FAT, LOSE WEIGHT AND
GAIN MUSCLE IN 12 WEEKS*

*FULL PRACTICE CUTTING PLAN, NUTRITION TIPS,
STRETCHES, EXTRA VEGAN INSIGHTS*

Disclaimer

Exercise is inherently strenuous and potentially dangerous. Consult your physician before starting any exercise program. Achilleas Karakatsanis is not responsible for injuries or health problems incurred as a result of exercise or related advice.

ISBN: 9781092945707

CONTENTS

Chapter One

The Flight Of Icarus

WHAT IS A CUTTING PROGRAM

AND WHY YOU SHOULD DO IT?

The reasons for cutting are simple. You have gained a few kilos from your previous training and now you want to cut those kilos and lose a good percentage of fat in the meantime. Unfortunately, whether we like it or not, we also gain fat when getting heavier with nutrition and training. We will also lose fat during cutting, but we will also lose muscle mass which we will get back with the training we will do every day.

Despite all this, you may be at the point where you have some extra weight and want to lose weight in general without any training rounds. You have gained weight from bad nutrition, lack of sleep and some bad habits in general, such as bad timing of your meals or the excessive size of your meals. On this matter, I will give you a piece of advice later that will significantly change the way you think about food.

Whichever may be the reason to lose weight, this is a cutting program that will help you set the right goals and accomplish them after the end of 12 weeks. You should devote yourself to your trainings but even more to your meals. Because if you don't have a negative balance (calorie deficit) on your total daily calories, then there is no way you will lose weight.

A negative calorie balance will help you lose weight slowly and steadily and with the trainings you will help your muscles grow and help burn fat during your day.

The cutting program refers mainly to your diet and your training style. The most important of all is your diet. Your calories should be less than what your body consumes in a rest state.

The second thing that contributes to cutting are your trainings. They are intense trainings that increase and decrease the heartrate to keep burning calories to maintain its energy. This is achieved by training.

With aerobic training (cardio) (treadmill, bike, HIIT, LISS) we achieve improved cardiovascular function to tolerate more intensity in our trainings so that we put out more intensity over time (progressive overload). Everything is connected.

Do not forget that!

So, to become Icarus, fly high and reach the sun, you have to lose the extra weight, put on muscle mass and cut. This way you will help your wings more so as to withstand your weight and fly for longer and higher!

Icarus set high goals and achieved them, but he missed the important thing of limits and moderation.

Because, as in bad habits, so in good ones, we must apply limits and moderation, otherwise they turn against us.

Anything good without limit and moderation can be fatal for our health or for the people around us. Take the example of Icarus and fly high to reach the Goals but do not let selfishness (ego-lifting) and arrogance take you down!

Now it's time to talk about some nice terms you need to know about the trainings you will be doing from us, but also some general terms you need to know to do your workouts better.

Let's go then

Mind - muscle connection:

With this term, we mean the communication your mind has with the muscle you're training as you train. It's a difficult technique that will take time, but in time you will understand that it helps a lot to target the weight of exercise exactly to the muscle you want.

A good technique used by Professional Bodybuilders for many years now and succeeds in its purpose is Posing. They sit in front of the mirror and tighten the muscles they will train and exercise in general.

This is an excellent technique that helps them understand which body movement and which joints strain the specific muscles.

They do not just like looking at the mirror and showing off their muscles. There is a technique behind all of this! Use it and see how your body reacts to each training session.Mechanical tension:

With this term we mean the intensity that a muscle group receives from the exercise we perform. How long we perform an exercise or how many repetitions (REPS) we do for a particular muscle group. In this technique the DropSet and SuperSet protocols help a lot. They train the muscle for a longer time, and so we achieve a greater protein synthesis in that muscle. Certainly, all this takes time.

This doesn't mean that if all of our exercises were dropset & superset in each Set then we would have seen a huge difference from the first week. The opposite seems to be the case.

Overtraining has the opposite effects of what we need. This means Hypertrophy.

Muscle-Damage:

This term refers to the damage the muscle receives as we perform a certain exercise. This technique uses longer duration of negative reps but also stretches the range of motion all the way to the top or bottom of the movement depending on the exercise.

What you actually do is you perform the concentric contraction in 1 second and the eccentric contraction (negative) in 3 to 5 seconds. Some athletes perform the Negative in more seconds but it depends on your level of experience.

This technique I almost the same with the Negatives Technique with the difference that the Negatives are more easy for a beginner to perform than the Muscle-Damage. Do not perform too many SETS of this technique cause you'll be more sore the next days. 1-2 sets is best according to your training protocol.

This way, we maintain tension in the muscle for longer, and so more muscle fibers are destroyed and we make the muscle withstand more intensity in the next training. While with the above we want to make it more resilient to Lactic Acid, in this technique we want to make it more tolerant to the intensity of exercise. That is, in the weight we put to perform the exercise.

Progressive Overload:

This term is used to define how much we want to progress each week in the exercises we do. In essence, this is also the purpose of exercising. Become stronger with the passing of time. Because in this way we ensure muscular Hypertrophy – that is Bulk. Each week we must progress 1.5% -2.5% from the previous week in kg or perform the same exercise with the same weight but more repetitions or, depending on the workout, to perform the exercise more quickly if the progress factor is time. In our case it's kilos. The aim of progressivity is to perform the exercise with more kilos per week, but to do so with both the correct technique and the same repetitions.

If you feel that you cannot perform all of the repetitions with the same technique and comfort as before, it's better to reduce weight. If for some reason you are pressured and you can't go on, you reverse the result.

Negatives:

This technique is mainly used in exercises that are very difficult to perform as beginners but also as moderate athletes. Some exercises such as pull ups are difficult regardless the experience of the athlete. We need years of training to be able to perform these exercises with comfort.

What we are doing is to start the exercise from the end of the Concentric contraction and to do the eccentric repeat as slowly as we can. For example, in the bar, we push with our feet to raise the head above the bar and from there we begin to descend downwards slowly. When we do negative repetitions, we exercise the same muscle groups as those during concentric contraction.

The same can be done in unilateral exercises like biceps. We finish the repetitions set and continue with the weak hand for another 4-5 repetitions but only the negative portion of the movement. We raise the dumbbell up with our other hand and lower the weight firmly and steadily for 3-4 seconds.

Superset (SS):

This technique is mainly used in trainings that need to raise the pace of training and force us to burn more calories during the training. We want to basically "burn" a muscle at different degrees and make it more resistant to the Lactic Acid.

For this reason, these trainings are sometimes called "lactic training". They help our muscles withstand more in exercises of maximum effort.
Like a marathon. The Supersets use competing muscles in principal. So, back with chest, biceps with triceps, quadriceps with biceps femoris. And we can also perform two exercises focusing on different degrees of the same muscle as upper and lower thoracic or front with rear deltoid.

Dropset:

Dropset also helps withstand lactic acid more but also helps us for a specific muscle.
This muscle undergoes major intensity in the last exercise Set because we cut weight in half 2 times and sometimes 3 or 4 and push the muscle to its limits.

Thus, more muscle fibers are used and we help in the further synthesis of muscle protein but we also help in some way the muscle to withstand more in lactic training like Cross Training, Crossfit, HIIT etc.

Unilateral:

This technique helps us use both sides of our body separately. Some sides are stronger than the others and we have to understand which, so we can use the technique of negative repetitions at the end of the Set to strengthen the weaker muscle. Just remember that one side is not all strong and the other all weak.

For example: I have strong right biceps and triceps but weak left ones. But I have strong left quadriceps and weak right ones. Strong right calves and weak left ones, weak left buttocks and strong right ones.

For a great deal I am stronger on the right but sometimes our body stance in our everyday life makes us weaker in one side.

All of these can change from day to day and from training to training. You have to remember every time what muscles to exercise a little more (with the same weight you put on the strong side) to reduce the differences in your body.

HIIT (High Intensity Interval Training):

This is a technique that is used and refers to the way and the intensity of training. Basically, you run for 30 seconds and walk for 15. Repeat 10 times. If you are at a good level, you can repeat 15 times. Generally, do not prefer it after leg exercises. You are already tired, and you will burn your legs more and there is no reason.

After leg training you can do a simple fast walk with an incline of 3% -5% incline so you do not burn your legs further and enjoy it. Do not prefer a step machine. They use quads more and you'll regret it the next day!

LIIT (Lower Intensity Interval Training):

It's the same as before just that this time you are running less and resting the same as you have run or even a little more.

That's 20 seconds running and 20 seconds rest or even more for resting. In essence, it is for beginners or for children or for people with injuries or don't want to be injured by the above technique.
If you want to achieve the same results as HIIT then you will have to do twice as much, that is, about a couple of hours.

BB & DB:

There are two shortcuts that you will meet a lot in our training, and we want you to know exactly what they mean in order not to look around at the last moment, when what you have to do is train. BB = Barbell & DB = Dumbbell. They are often used in a lot of workouts out there so it's good to know what you are reading.

Overtrained:

Someone is considered Overtrained if they see little or no difference in their body over time while using the above 6 first techniques. This is due to a few factors that have to do with Overtraining of the athlete. This means that the athlete has exceeded some fine limits that he or she should not have, and the body can't keep up with the changes. In order for our body to function properly internally, you should:

1. Rest for 7 to 8 hours every night and sleep the necessary hours. I hope it is before 00.00 but if work does not allow that, then it would be good to sleep 7 to 8 hours a day. If work also does not allow that too, then try to keep the next.

2. Do not go for 7 out of 7 trainings a week and don't rest properly. After such intensity at the gym and such intensity in your daily life and work in general, your body needs more time to fully replenish what it "lost" during the training. And with the lack of time you're not helping it to do so properly and you stay the same even though you train a lot at the gym or any other workout place. Try to work out 4 times a week for 2 weeks and for the next two weeks to work out 5 times a week and then 6 and then 4 and 5 and so on.

3. Maybe your diet does not allow you to do the right recovery. You may not work and have time for sleeping and you still see no results. Then overtraining is due to a lack of dietary habits. However if you get used to eating

a home meal and the rest of it is takeaway and still be in the calories you want, then you may not eat so much or so little depending on your goal. In our case, you might think you eat less than you do, or even the same number of calories as your daily rest state. Consult a dietician and you will see how you will immediately see a difference.

All of this has nothing to do with our program, but they are good to know because you may find yourself in a similar situation at some point in your life and remember all that you have read here and help you with your, at the time, training and goals!

Last but not Least!

What we always say in all gyms and hardly anyone seems to understand! It's as if we do not even say it sometimes.

Re - Rack Your Weights and Accessories

It is not difficult to make the decision and put the barbells in their place. Take the weights off the bar and put them in their place. Remove the bars or handles from the pulleys and put them back in their place. Because guess what... someone else would want to use them after you.

Why find them as you left them? It's an important detail that makes the difference and helps the rest athletes in the gym. Because there exist not just the massive guys that can lift the whole building with one hand. Also registered are older people, women and children.

Don't show off with the barbells. Also have a towel with you, put on deodorant and do not sit on a machine with the mobile in hand! You are there to achieve your goals. Not to mess with your phone. Put it aside for the couple of hours you'll be there and enjoy the moment of your training.

That way you will be able to acquire this mind - muscle connection we mentioned above!
Before we start the journey of Cutting we have some things to discuss about.

The way to lose fat and build muscle is to follow a training plan for cutting with low resting periods between sets. Low as much as 30 seconds. 30 to 45 seconds is optimal for burning fat during your trainings. I don't promise its going to be faster but I guarantee it will be a better way to do it.

The other way is with Fasted Cardio. Let me explain a little further what I mean about Fasted and about Cardio.

Fasted means you haven't eat something the last 8 to 12 hours. So your stomach is empty and all your energy storages are full. So when you begin your Cardio session your body starts burning all energy supply from your liver and then from your muscles. Thats not a lot of energy if you consider that you're in a caloric deficit.

That means you eat less amounts of Carbohydrates (Carbs) and so you have less energy from Carbs to give for energy to your muscles. Something important to notice here. When you are in a carbohydrate deficit you might have pressure management issues.

That means you are getting upset more easily and you lose your temper. Be sure to control that cause its going to happen sometimes and you have to think its all about carbs. They help you maintain your energy but when your energy storages are off you are usually off control! Don't panic. Just be aware and control it!

So, the next sources of energy are protein and fat. Its the last two energy sources given to you when carbs are over. In about 20 minutes of cardio or weight training you have limited your carb sources of energy and your body will lead to protein and fat.

More blood is flowing because your Heart Rate is up and going and so more protein and fat will flow in you for energy.

Cardio can be hard, cruel, sad and/or depressing for some people. But it shouldn't be. Its a good way to lose fat and/or accumulate strength and endurance.

Its the most common way to achieve your endurance goals. And it's a way to see your body shine again. Feel your skin toned and your strength going all the way to the top.

While some people think its a way to lose fat only, I have to say that is a way to lift more weights also. Because if your Heart Rate can't support the effort your body and muscles are making for such a lift then you can't lift anything. If you struggle to lift maybe its because of poor Heart Rate capabilities.

Its a way to build bigger lifts and a way to lose fat and or muscle if you don't train properly.

So lets get things in order for you.
What you have to do when you cut is to enroll in your training 4 to 5 Cardio sessions and lots of walking, taking the stairs, parking away from your company or house.

Cardio is not found only in the gym. Its an everyday task we can enroll in our everyday life.

What you have to do is simple. Either you do an Interval Training, or a steady Cardio Session.

A fast walk outside or a moderate walk on the Treadmill with an incline of 10% to 14%. Until you reach 40 minutes.

Also you can do a whole steady Cardio Session of 40 minutes. On a moderate pace with 8% to 14% incline.
By Moderate I mean a speed where you can talk to someone but you can't talk like when you're just standing.

Everything in the Fitness Industry is simple. But by all means nothing is easy as it might seems. Everything you do needs time, effort and some sacrifices. Your most valuable would be TIME.

You have to give at least 10 to 12 hours at least per week to achieve your Fitness Goals. That is 4 to 5 trainings and 4 to 6 Cardio Sessions per week. Its the least you can do to achieve something in only 12 weeks and do it well.

And as I said above everything is simple because the Marketing Industry of Fitness and Nutrition makes it seem difficult.

So you can buy their products and services so you can achieve something faster and 'smarter'.

But if you think you're smarter than the other then think again.

You better give your TIME than waste your hard earned money on products that work better with the PLACEBO EFFECT.

If you don't know about it then you just Google it.

Fat Loss is slower in the Kitchen and Faster on the Gym

Its not so difficult to do it.
It just takes time to learn about your Macros and how many calories each food and snack has.

Educate Yourself and make your Fitness Journey easier.
Better safe than sorry.
You don't have to lose money and your precious time to achieve half the results and start over again.

Or maybe you won't start again because you'll think that a Fit Life is just not for you.

Well, you're wrong. Its for everyone. You just have to follow the right paths and not the easy paths.

A SUM OF ALL THE ABOVE IS

- TRAINING = 4 to 6x/WEEK

- RESTING PERIOD = 30 to 45 seconds between SETS

- CARDIO SESSIONS = INTERVAL TRAINING AND/OR STEADY CARDIO

- INTERVAL TRAINING = 30 sec run followed by 30 sec active rest (walking) for 10 to 15 times.

- STEADY CARDIO = 40 mins of FAST WALKING WITH INCLINE OF 10% to 14%.

- FIRST INTERVAL THEN STEADY FOR THE REMAINING 40 mins OR

- ONLY STEADY CARDIO FOR 40 mins.

Before you begin your workouts we have included an important list from our previous book to help you through your practice

- Any muscle imbalances you may have in your body, such as your biceps (right or left), either in your legs or arms, you can correct, so both look the same. You cannot change how the muscle fibres are formed inside your body, but you can change a different looking arm or leg. You can do that by always begin with your weaker part first. After you finish the SET you perform another 4-5 reps with the imbalanced muscle. That way you help your muscle to grow and look like the other one. It will take time and effort. Don't wait immediate results.

• R E L A X. Do your workouts, keep the right nutrition and everything will be fine.

• Remember to be consistent in your training and nutrition.

• Be strong and smile every day. In essence, from here on that's how you'll be. Exercising elevates the levels of testosterone, the growth hormone and endorphins and because of that you are happier and more active in your day.

• Learn to be consistent and true to your goals, otherwise you will not see the results you expect. An average waiting time is 6 months. 6 months of good workouts, balanced nutrition and good rest is equivalent to many beautiful effects on your body and spirit.

• Always log the weights you lift. We have created a separate cell next to set and reps so you can log the kilos/ pounds you lift for each exercise. The best would be to note how much you lifted on the first set and how much on the last one. It is very important to note your weights so that your help yourself do a proper progressive overload in weights every week. This is achieved with a 2.5% added weight per week per exercise. So don't forget to note down your kilos on the form we have created.

- Sleep for 7 to 9 hours. We have said this many times and we will keep saying it. Because sleep is the biggest anabolic in hypertrophy. Insufficient levels of sleep mean our body does not get the chance to make up for the injured cells that were lost during the training and the next day we will not have progressed as much as we should. Be consistent. Once more. Be consistent. Think of your future self. That way, you will be able to move forward, even when you want to stay in your house.

- Stretch before and after. Dynamic stretching before training that mimic the movements of the exercises you will do without or with light weights. Also, static stretching at the end of the trainings for better muscle recovery over the next few days. Below we have included some stretches with illustrations and explanations.

- Watch videos, read articles from us and from other pages and be informed on what you're doing. Always have a more general image of the things you occupy yourself with. It's good for your workouts, but more importantly for yourself.

- Remember that CARDIO is important but in the right way. This mentality of endless hours on the treadmill, circuit programs and high-intensity training with minimal breaks was a sort of marketing from a bygone era that never seems to go away. You have to understand that Cardio helps you lose fat while you're doing it. And it does not need to be in great intensity. Moderate-intensity walking with a low or high incline (depending on how much your knees can take) is enough to do the job. On the other hand, resistance training (weight training) make the body burn fat while not in the gym. In short terms, that is. The compound exercises (squats, deadlifts, hip thrusts, chest presses, shoulder presses, rowing, etc.) use a lot of muscles in our body and in this way, more muscles stay on alert and the body learns to be on alert until the next training. And that's why we burn fat while we're out of the gym.

We thought it would be nice to give you some information about the 7 Compound movements we practice the most.

SEVEN BASIC COMPOUND MOVEMENTS EXPLAINED

Its the basic movements every trained or untrained athlete will use when hitting the gym, a crosfit gym or at any weightlifting workout.

These compound movements are the basis of all because by applying them and analysing the movement of the muscles involved the exercises progressed through isolation movements such as bicep curls, tricep curls, leg extensions, leg curls, walking lunges, lateral raises, shrugs.

All these movements came along after the compound movements because athletes and or coaches wanted to train a specific muscle.

Like train the lats and biceps for someone who's sport is rowing. All of these exercises are both for strength and hypertrophy.

1. BARBELL SQUAT:

They target the thigh muscles, hips and glutes. Quadriceps (all four heads) as well as hamstrings and also ligaments and the bones. Its also a good exercise to work your core because you have to balance all the weight with your core. It is also a Powerlifting Lift.

You can Squat with a Barbell, Dumbbells, Kettlebells and Cables and/or Bands.

2. DEADLIFT:

The first letter of the phrase (DEAD) is referred to the movement. Which means that you start the movement without momentum.

That means Dead-starting point. The muscles included are too much to refer to but I will inform you with the basic.

Gluteus (Maximus, minimus), bicep femurs (one head of the hamstrings) and semitendinosus, and semimembranosus (the other head of hamstrings). It is also a Powerlifting Lift.

You can Deadlift with a Barbell, Dumbbells, Kettlebells.

3. BARBELL CHEST PRESS:

They target the pectoralis major muscle, as well as anterior deltoids, serratus anterior, coracobrachialis, and the triceps. Wider Grip is associated with training the pecs and narrowed Grip with Triceps (Close Grip Press).

It uses the core for stabilisation (transverse abdominis, obliques, erector spinae).

It's the best exercise to build strength and muscle on the pecs. The first movement was the Floor Press. It is also a Powerlifting Lift.

You can Chest Press with a Barbell, Dumbbells, Kettlebells, Bands and Chains.

And the variations include Incline and Decline Bench Press, Landmine Press, Cable Crossover.

4. BARBELL OVERHEAD PRESS:

They target the anterior deltoids and there is some involvement of the pecs and also the trapezius muscle.

There are lots of Variations to this exercise such as Arnold Press (named after Arnold Schwarzenegger), Behind-the-neck-Press, Bradford Press (as you pass your head with the bar you slowly pass the bar behind the neck and then explosively pass the bar over your head to the front and slowly to the starting position),

Dumbbell Press, Military Press (stiff legs with no pushing movement from legs), Olympic Clean and Press, Unilateral Press, Push Press (using leg drive to press the barbell up), seated Press and Sots Press (Pressing the Barbell up from a deep squat position. Named after Viktor Sots).

You can Shoulder Press with a Barbell, Dumbbells, Kettlebells, Bands.

5. PULL UPS:

Target the pulling muscles such as arms (biceps brachii), shoulders (teres major especially the posterior muscles), rhomboids and trapezius muscles, Pectoralis major and minor.

The abdominal muscles stabilize the movement (external and internal obliques).

The forearms also create an isometric contraction during the movement. Some variations are Weighted, Mixed Grip, One Arm and One Hand-the difference is that One hand is easier because with one hand you hold the grip and with the other you grip the other arm below the wrist-, Kipping, Muscle-Up, Chin Up and Inverted Row.

6. BARBELL BENTOVER ROW:

Target the latissimus dorsi muscle, trapezius, posterior deltoids, infraspinatus and teres minor.

The movement also targets the core as it stabilizes the movement. Maintaining an arch during the movement will help you lift the weights and also maintain a healthy lower back.

Some variations of the movement are T-Bar Rows, Dumbbell Rows, Pendley Rows (explosively pull the bar to your chest and let it drop to the floor immediately after reaching top, then Repeat again), Rowing Machine (not chest supported), Underhand Grip Row, One arm bent-over dumbbell row.

7. BARBELL HIP THRUSTS:

Target the gluteus Maximus and hamstrings too. But there is more muscle involvement in hip thrusts rather than squats. The load is more on the hips rather than the spine.

Find the best position for you with the knees and hip make 90 degreed angle. If you put your feet wider or narrower you target other areas.

And if you place your feet closer to your glutes you target more hamstrings.

Find your right spot cause its different for some people. Its that mind-muscle connection that makes the difference.

Compound Movements Alternative Exercises

For any injured muscles or trainees who cannot yet do these exercises:

Back Squats:

Walking Lunges, goblet squats (front squats), side squats, Bulgarian Split Squats, Split Squats (close stance=quads / wide stance=gluteus), Jump Squats(plyo), Box Jumps, Step-Ups (lean forward more quadriceps focused).

Deadlifts:

Rack Pulls, Dumbbell Deadlifts, Straight Arms Pulldowns, Pullover, Romanian Deadlifts w/ wide feet, Assisted Heavy Dumbbell Bentover Row

Military Press:

Shoulder Press + Machine, Front Raises with hands externally rotated (means your thumbs pointing up), lateral raises.

I won't put any cable exercise because it gives too much tension on the shoulders at whole range of motion.

Chest Press:

Dumbbell Chest Press, Landmine Press, Dips, Dumbbell Flys, Push Ups, Peck Deck, Push Ups Machine.

We won't put any cable exercise because it gives too much tension on the shoulders at whole range of motion.

Pull Ups or Inverted Rows:

Cable Rows, Lat Pulldowns, Chin-downs, Barbell or Dumbbell Bentover Rows, Machine Rows, Shrugs and Pullover, Straight Arms Pulldowns, Rear Delts w/ cable or Dumbbell.

BARBELL Bent Overhand or Underhand Row:

Rear Delts w/ cable or Dumbbell, Shrugs and machine Row, T-Bar, Pendley Rows, Dumbbell Bentover Rows, Single Arm Rows, V-Grip Pulldowns

BARBELL Hip Thrusts:

Cable Pull Throughs, kettlebell dumbbell swings, glute bridge w/dumbbell, side or lying kicks w/ cable, leg press upper feet stance, Glute Kicks w/ cable, fire hydrants, walking lunges w/ wide stance.

If you don't know any of these, you can look them up online. We apologize for not describing these exercises, but it is because we wanted our book to be small and inclusive.

So, if you are in this category then what you have to do due to anatomy is exercises where you can stand and perform standing.

This way you stress your back less, because the weight is put on your legs and in the limbs you press with. When you have bent knees and hips, the energy passes through your entire body and does not stop in any "locked" joint, simply put.

When sitting, virtually all the weight falls into your back and you stress it more while thinking that you help your situation.

On the contrary, you're worsening it. Remember this the next time you do an exercise.

Chapter Two

Macronutrients and Dietary Supplements

Introduction to the Components of a Balanced Nutrition and Training

This chapter is transferred from our other book titled "Your Personal Hypertrophy Workout Plan", which aims to increase the muscle volume (bulking). This information does not change due to training but remain the same in every type of training you do. We have added an extra portion to this book on Nutrition for Vegetarians.

DIETARY SUPPLEMENTS:

You take supplements if you cannot have food ready from home. If you manage to have a balanced diet, then you do not need more protein in a Shake. You will need creatine and omega-3 fat, zma (B12, zinc and magnesium) and a lot of water when you reach a satisfactory level.

In the winter when I start my bulk trainings because I have free time and I can cook, I take no protein supplements.

Only some of the ones I will mention below. When my macronutrients are complete, I don't need to 'load' my body with more protein. Besides, when you want to put on weight you have to increase your carbohydrates and fats relative to protein. Protein is 1.4-1.8g per kilos of bodyweight, the carbohydrates is 4-4.2g, and the fats is 1.2-1.5g.

You do not need to study much more of them, but to be consistent and disciplined towards training, nutrition and above all, yourself. Remember that your health comes before your image in the mirror and the weights you want to lift with your arms or chest or legs.

Let's put them in order in your mind.

PROTEIN:

4 CALORIES PER GRAM.

The most widespread supplement and perhaps the most mythical one. You get a protein Shake and you just become huge.

Veins pumping from everywhere, your chest or butt pops out and you are ready to destroy the entire gym with your power. And suddenly you take protein before training and your workouts are the same!

You take some every time before and after but you don't become huge. Maybe it's the brand's fault. I'll find another.

But you forget something very important: protein is a macronutrient that helps build the muscle fibers 'injured' by training. It is also a good source of energy for your workouts if you manage to "burn" all the glycogen stores on your liver and muscles. Which in their entirety is 500 gr.

With 4 calories per 1g, carbohydrates alone in our body account for 2000 calories. A lot, right? However, they are needed to provide us with all the movements we do every day.

Not just to lift in the gym, but also climb the stairs, walk, lift groceries, open a door, move our hands or feet, etc., but let me continue on the protein...

A basic macronutrient ingredient that contributes to the good functioning of our muscles and also to our _better_ recovery.

Watch out! _Better_, not faster! No supplement does wonders, because it's simply a "supplement". It's a food substitute. They are not performance enhancing drugs or androgens.

So, we need protein right after training so it can do its job of repairing the injured muscles.

And in the remaining meals until we sleep, we need more carbohydrates and protein at the same level (40g-60g/meal).

CARBOHYDRATES:

4 CALORIES PER GRAM.

Carbohydrates are the most important source of energy in our bodies. When we deal with anything in our daily lives that changes the length of our muscles, we consume carbohydrates from the liver's stores (first store) and then the muscle glycogen (second store).

That's why it's important to have a good amount of carbohydrates in our diet. Carbohydrates are among the most important macronutrients because they contribute to the smooth functioning of the muscles and most of our body's functions.

FATS:

9 CALORIES PER GRAM.

Fat, besides fat around the waist, also contributes as a thermostat to our body. With fat, water and blood the temperature of our body is regulated. With fat we also draw energy for our workouts when glycogen stores run out.

It is good to have a percentage around 10% to 16% in our body when we want to gain muscle weight but also when we want to lose weight. In essence, when we gain weight we will put on lean mass as well as fat.

It is inevitable. Just as when we lose weight, we lose both fat and muscular mass. Just with the right diet and exercise we will keep it at the rates it was before, until the end of our workouts.

HYDRATION:

1 TO 2 LITRES PER DAY.

Water is a very important factor in both sports and nutrition. The greatest percentage in our body as well as in our muscles is water. For this reason, we need to drink enough water to be hydrated throughout our day and during our workouts.

For this reason, we also need to consume sodium (salt). Because salt does fluid retention in our body and uses it when our body needs it.

To give you a picture of your muscles I will explain what they have inside:

- Protein (18%)
- Fat (5%)
- Carbohydrates (1%)
- Vitamins and minerals (1%)
- Water (75%)

Therefore, we understand that water is very important for our training as well as for our body in general. It also helps as perform better our workouts.

If we are dehydrated we will perform poor. Below we have a table that helps you learn how much water you need according to your weight:

So, per 5 kilos of bodyweight, we add 0.2 liter of water per day.

ALCOHOL AND JUNK FOOD:

7 and 9 CALORIES PER GRAM.

Alcohol and junk food contain the most calories. That's why it's reasonable to have junk food or a drink once a week. Apart from the fact that the macronutrients of junk food are deficient in terms of quality (protein, fiber) and too much in terms of fats, simple and complex carbohydrates. The protein they contain is minimal or equal sometimes but not of the same biological value. That way, our body absorbs much less macronutrients because it does not recognize the ingredients that fall into our stomach.

That's why much caution is needed when we eat out. We may need to eat more some days (1-2 times a week) but it would be good to be careful what we EAT.

OMEGA 3 AND 6 FATS:

MICRONUTRIENTS.

Omega 3 and 6 fatty acids help your body and especially the muscles to recover better. Not faster, _better_! Omega fats are known to provide better muscle performance and recovery. They also help with brain function and better performance of our immune system. For this, it is important to eat fatty fish foods. If you don't have the time to cook fish, then an omega 3 or 6 supplement would be very good for your diet.

Within 10 days you will see the difference on how your body responds after the training and the following days. Your feet or back may hurt the day after training but remember, that's a good sign. Three (3) capsules per day is the recommended dose and should not be exceeded. One capsule after your meal.

CREATINE*:

Creatine or phosphocreatine is the body's fuel during the first 10 seconds of exercise. It increases performance by 10-15% on single or repeated short (up to 30 seconds) maximum efforts. It is the fastest form of 'fuel' since it is consumed very quickly but it brings a lot of energy to our muscles. For this reason, a supplement of creatine is important. Which is the purest supplement on the market right now. Nothing bad happens if you take it and our body absorbs it right away. But we need to take it because we can't store too much.

5g per day before the training is enough to give you explosiveness between sets and to help you fill up your energy in less time than the one indicated in each training session. It is such a pure supplement that does not need either 'charging' or loading circles. You can start and stop it immediately. Professional bodybuilders stop it when they are in a weight losing period because the creatine hydrates our muscles.

Because water in performance and in the recovery of muscles is very important. And surely these athletes do not want a hint of water on their bodies during the days of the contest. It has an anabolic effect (muscle growth) when combined with strength training. Also, possible injury prevention and improved immune function exist. So, let's learn from the example.

*No serious side effects from long-term use have been reported.

MULTIVITAMINS:

Multivitamins are suggested to people who can't manage to get their vitamins from food and do not get to eat fruits and vegetables.

Once a day is enough to contribute to good concentration and increase our energy levels.

1 to 2 capsules depending on our nutritional needs.

ZMA:

Zma is a vitamin supplement with zinc, magnesium and vitamin B12. All three offer better recovery of injured muscle fibers while resting in our sleep. They greatly contribute to the proper functioning of our organs, our immune system and our bones. 2-3 capsules 2 hours before sleep on an empty stomach. Do not consume dairy products before zma, as they break down vitamin function.

Your Weight	Liters of Water per Day
45	1.9
50	2.1
55	2.3
60	2.5
65	2.7
70	2.9
75	3.1
80	3.3
85	3.5

BRANCH-CHAINED AMINO ACIDS (BCAAS):

Bcaas are the essential amino acids leucine, isoleucine, valine. The combination of these amino acids makes up about 1/3 of the skeletal muscle tissue.

After training, the bcaas put the body in an increased hypertrophic state by increasing protein composition. Bcaas are metabolized within the muscle cell and not in the liver.

This means they are more likely to be used for muscle synthesis than as a fuel for energy.

FRUIT AND VEGETABLES:

It is important to eat fruit and vegetables because they give us their vitamins and their plant fibers.

Besides that, they help us with our cravings for sweets and keeps our stomach full for at least a while.

Fruit consumption is suggested one hour before eating and not after, because the fructose contained in them makes digestion after a meal difficult.

Vegetables should be consumed in our meals as follows:

- In the bulk phase we eat our meal and then the vegetables or somewhat along with the meal.

- In the weight loss phase, we eat vegetables first and then our meal.

- Vegetables, because of the fibers and the carbohydrates contained in them, make us feel fuller.

- In the phase we are now, we consume our vegetables after or alongside our lunch and fruits before our meal or after training.

REST:

Rest is one of our most important priorities in our workouts and muscle hypertrophy.

It helps to recover muscles injured during training and to redistribute energy stores in our body until the next training. The more rested we are, the more efficient we will be and the more we will benefit from muscle hypertrophy.

Maybe you don't understand how important it is now, but in the long run you will realise that without rest we cannot have beautiful results. Everything must be in harmony to have better results. You can't do a little of everything and get the best results. You can't eat a little and expect to be full.

Just as you can't eat a lot and expect to lose weight. Just remember how important resting and sleeping 7 to 9 hours a day is:

- Faster recovery of our muscles.

- Increased levels of testosterone and growth hormone.

- More energy for your workouts.

- Sleep reduces cortisol levels in our body.

But let's talk about what you're thinking.

What is this cortisol? Surely, it's not some bug spray.

In a few words, cortisol is the hormone of anxiety. It causes many problems in our body with some of them being the following:

- loss of muscle mass

- weakening of our immune system

- Hyperglycaemia

- In large proportions it leads to minimal wound healing

Cortisol is essential for our body to produce epinephrine. However, when produced in large proportions, it has very bad effects on our body.

So, it's good to try to keep it under control as much as we can.

MEAL FREQUENCY:

Big issue, I know! The frequency of meals is something that depends on the person. During the day you have a calorie limit to consume. Let's say 2000 calories. The least would be in 4 meals. From then on, you can have as many meals as you want or whatever makes you feel full throughout your day. For example, I do 7 to 8 meals a day.

Arnold Schwarzenegger did 5 meals a day when he wanted to gain weight. The amount of meals you do depends on your appetite and whether it keeps you full during the day. So, there is no right and wrong.

Just remember to eat a regular meal 2-3 hours before training or fruit and protein 1-2 hours before and after training to take your protein and have a meal 1-2 hours after that. So set your diet right around your workouts, and then see how your body reacts to the meals of the day.

At least 4 meals during the day if you want to get good results. And one after your training. Not immediately after it. Let one hour pass and then eat your meal.

FREQUENCY OF TRAINING:

The best for last! Workout frequency has to do with how many times you want to train your muscle groups.

The best is to train each muscle group twice a week.

That way, we contribute more to muscle hypertrophy and we have better results. In our program we have combined at least 5 trainings in the hypertrophy weeks and 3-4 trainings per week for strength weeks.

Strength is important for hypertrophy because it makes us stronger so we can lift more in the weeks of hypertrophy, in a few wise words.

The best training protocol is 6 days a week with the two training sessions being strength.

4 to 6 workouts per week.

HOW TO BE A VEGETARIAN

Not everything around us becomes weird, it is just that people react negatively to change in general. Sometimes we have to learn better about what's going on around us and not just listen to what those who accuse them have to say about them.

It's not something bad, and it's certainly not something that goes unnoticed. And for it to go on for so long it means that it is something that deserves our effort because it concerns people and the rest of the living beings on this planet.

This is not a book that focuses on researching this issue and for this reason I will not talk about why it started and when but how you can change your diet with plant products rather than dairy and animal products.

The only thing I can say as a result is that a person who stops eating animal products and their byproducts as well as dairy and eggs helps to save:

1100 gallons of water*
45 lbs. of grain
30 sq. ft forest
10lbs of CO_2
1 animal

*Source: Cowspiracy - The sustainability secret

All this is needed in the meat, dairy and egg production factories to produce their products for one day from a single animal. I know very well that this is a chapter that may not interest many readers, but it is good to have an in-depth knowledge of our real world. It is good to learn and evolve around the issues that concern both training and nutrition. Our ancestors lived longer because of nutrition and not some magical phenomenon or for less atmospheric pollution.

Vegetarianism is the practice of abstaining from the consumption of meat (red meat, poultry, seafood, and the flesh of any other animal), and may also include abstention from by-products of animal slaughter.

Some reviews have shown that some people who eat vegan diets have less chronic disease, including heart disease, than people who do not follow a restrictive diet.

Ancient Greek philosophy has a long tradition of vegetarianism. Pythagoras was reportedly vegetarian (and studied at Mt. Carmel, where some historians say there was a vegetarian community), as his followers were expected to be.

Roman writer Ovid concluded his magnum opus Metamorphoses, in part, with the impassioned argument (uttered by the character of Pythagoras) that in order for humanity to change, or metamorphose, into a better, more harmonious species, it must strive towards more humane tendencies.

He cited vegetarianism as the crucial decision in this metamorphosis, explaining his belief that human life and animal life are so entwined that to kill an animal is virtually the same as killing a fellow human.

Source:
https://en.wikipedia.org/wiki/Vegetarianism#Classical_Greek_and_Roman_philosophy

It is good to do research first and then go on to doing anything. When we start something, especially something so subversive in our lives, it is good to start slowly.

We should not think of what we will go through by changing a habit in our life, but what that will bring to us in the end. Better living, a healthier relationship with our body and the environment.

The beginning is always the hardest, but we have to start somewhere.

And I fall into this case because I have to learn to eat less and less animal foods.

I was eating almost every day. But now I'm trying to eat as little animal products as possible. It is a good opportunity for your body to detoxify and test something different.

Do not make the change abruptly.

We will give you advice on what foods to eat and you will start if you want to. What we want you to do is slowly shift.

Some foods that you can choose in your diet when you don't want to eat meat, or its products are as follows:

SESAME SEEDS	OATS	KIDNEY BEANS	BANANAS	HEMP SEEDS
BROCCOLI	SPINACH	SWEET POTATOES	POTATOES	KALE
TOFU	CARROTS	GARLIC	TOMATOES	PEANUTS
CUCUMBER	ORANGES	PEAS	RICE	PASTA
BREAD	PEARS	BULGUR WHEAT	PEANUT BUTTER	CHICKPEAS
HUMMUS	ONIONS	TOMATO SAUCE	90% DARK CHOCOLATE	COCONUT
BRAN FLAKES	WEETABIX	PRUNES	CASHEWS	ALMONDS
BLUEBERRIES	MANGO	GARBANZO BEANS	TAHINI	LENTILS

Worldwide, the products for Vegetarians have increased their production by 60%.

While worldwide sales of vegetarian products are increasing every year by 24%.

Below is a table of basic foods corresponding to macronutrients

Vegan Macros:

Protein:

Lentils, Chickpeas & beans of every kind, Tempeh, Tofu, Seitan, Nutritional Yeast, Chlorella, rice/hemp protein powders,

Fats:

Avocado, chia seeds, flaxseeds, nuts, dark chocolate, peanut butter and other nut butters, cacao nibs, olive

Carbs:

Fruit, potatoes, oats, rice, quinoa and whole grains, veggies, legumes.

CHAPTER THREE

DAILY CALORIE INTAKE

INTRODUCTION TO THE COMPONENTS OF A BALANCED NUTRITION AND TRAINING

WHY YOU CAN'T LOSE WEIGHT AND/OR FAT?

WHAT MATTERS IS THE GOAL

WHAT DO YOU WANT TO ACHIEVE AT THE END OF OUR WORKOUTS?

THIS IS A PROGRAM TO LOSE FAT AND GAIN LEAN MUSCLE MASS THROUGH COMPOUND MOVEMENTS AND ACCESSORIES EXERCISES

WITH MORE FOCUS ON TRAINING TECHNIQUES SUCH AS SUPERSETS AND DROPSETS

First of all, consult a dietician to get you a proper diet plan. You can tell him what foods you like, what supplements and vitamins you consume daily to know exactly how to create your diet. If you do not want to see a dietician, my advice is to eat every single meal until you feel 80% full (this means the 4-5 mouthfuls before completing your meal) and at one big meal go for 100% full.

In this period the best you can do is to focus your meals around protein and vegetables. Carbohydrates should be reduced in half or even less sometimes depending on the content of your meal.

A good alternative is to eat a cup of cottage cheese together with half your lunch when you do not want to eat too much. You can eat a single cup as a meal. But I believe that in order to get to know when you are 80% full, you have to spend a lot of time with enough diets and analyses in your mind to understand your eating habits.

So, if you start now, a nutritionist is the best choice. Invest the money to get you a diet for 2 months and then combine those he gives you to change your meals and not eat the same all the time.

Something very important.

Do not worry or panic. We all started from scratch at some point in our life. No one knew "what" and "how" from the beginning.

This is nice at times. Because you learn yourself from the beginning and become better. You react to certain diets, foods, trainings, challenges in general.

This way you learn how to reach your Goals better every time. Do a meta-analysis of your week on Saturday or Sunday concerning your diet so you can understand what you did wrong and not make the same mistakes next time. Discipline and Courage is needed, and everything will be done.

So, let's continue with the next.
Download an application and start recording the food you eat for breakfast, lunch and dinner. This will help you get a sense of the number of calories in proportion to their weight for the foods you choose daily for your diet. The rates given to you (grams or lbs) by the nutritionist for each day correspond to certain foods and these foods correspond to certain calories.

Learn how many calories they have. That way, you will know the number of calories you eat, even when you have no scale. The only thing that is difficult to measure calories for is takeaway food and desserts. Typically, it's about 1.4 the normal calories. Sometimes more or even twice.

A very important detail to look for while losing weight is to remember to measure the areas in your body with the most fat.

From there you can see if you are actually losing weight and actually losing fat.

And also, do not weigh yourself once a week. A lot of changes happen in our body during the week and maybe one day you will have fluid retention and the scale will show 500 grams more and get you lost in the chaos of your thoughts and that day or the next you may eat far less than you should. This is not the right way. You will weigh yourself every day at the same time or at least 3 to 4 times a week. And at the end of the month you will divide this number by the times you measured yourself to get the average you need.

Do not worry too much with the numbers you see. Sometimes anxiety and sadness change the composition of our body and produce different numbers. That does not mean that we have certainly made a mistake in our diet or in our exercise. This means that we have to think reasonably and that we need to see the bigger picture.

Which is our image in 3 months that we will have finished our training and nutrition plan. The aim is to get through this as calm and cool as possible. Do not panic when something goes wrong.

Remember that all of this is part of the game and that in order to make a change properly you have to spend time and effort.

But do not ruin your progress with negative thoughts and worry that what you do has no effect or that you are doing it wrong.

The complexity of our body is immense, and we cannot always understand why some changes happen, but we must become more patient so that we can continue every day and see the results we need.

As for the whole fat thing I mentioned in the title. Let me point out that different people have fat in different areas in their bodies.

And to note something else: <u>you can't lose fat from a particular area of your body because you just do a certain exercise.</u> And the most common example here is the fat in the abdomen and people who do thousands of crunches and sit-ups to lose fat there.

The body does not focus on the exercise you perform, but on the stress it feels in its whole. It raises metabolism, burns through its energy stores and tries to respond to this moment. So, it burns fat and energy from everywhere.

Do not listen to diets and exercises that offer quick results.

If you expect quick results, then you will have a quick reset to your previous state.

Do not believe all these quick results theories. It's as if you just got your driver's license with zero experience on the road and drive a Ferrari with nitro. And at the first turn you push every pedal. Guess in how many seconds you will disappear from the face of the Earth...

Only you can do this with the hard work you will do in your trainings but even more in your diet. Because this is a cutting program and you have to focus your attention on the food!

Do not stray from your goal and do not wish for it to come faster. It will happen in its time and you will have gotten the biggest lesson from it.

To know yourself better.
How to eat properly and how to exercise properly! We will live with ourselves until the day we die, and we have to learn it very well so that we can give it all it deserves and even more!

Listen to yourself and make a step to achieve your goals from now on!

Do not leave anything for tomorrow.
The only thing we have to work on is today and this is the most beautiful part!

Because from today you can build a more beautiful future and live as you have always dreamt it!

One last thing.

Things you do not look after in your everyday life

1. How fast you eat your meals. It is very important to give our attention to our meals so that we can assimilate their ingredients better. It would be very good to have no screen in front of us while we eat (except for rare exceptions due to work or our beloved person). Unfortunately, we have not realized how important our lunch is. Every meal we have in the day and do not give it the necessary attention. As important as it is for us to take a break for 10 minutes and look at the sky or think about nothing to ease up, it's even more important to pay attention to our meal and how we chew our food. The more chewed the food gets to the stomach, the better we digest it and the more it will fill us during the day. Also, when we chew fast, we swallow air, and this also inflates our stomach without food and also makes us burp for the rest of the hour or day. Put aside the phone and the laptop and devote 10 to 15 minutes to enjoy your meal and you will see that in a few days you will enjoy your meal and every taste of it more and you will feel full for more hours. That way you will also find out when you are 80% full and stop

your meal so you can achieve your goal of losing weight and strengthening your body better.

2. How much water you consume during the day. It is very important to hydrate your body with water because water helps with most of our vital functions. Besides that, I want you to remember that when you are dehydrated, you cannot concentrate, and you cannot do your training properly. The muscles are not hydrated and do not reach their full capacity, so you struggle and strain yourself more than what it needs. It is very important to drink water. One to two sips every hour will offer you all the amount of water you need to feel more energetic during the day. And I will give you a little hint that will help you a lot. The bladder is adjustable. Which means that when we drink less water it is adjusted and reduced in size and strength. This simply means that when we start drinking more water and go to the toilet more, it does not mean that you do not need to drink any more water, but that the capacity of the bladder is met more frequently and needs immediate evacuation. After 2-3 weeks it will grow, and you will be able to withstand more water consumption and adapt to the new amount of water you consume. So don't think you've drank as much as you needed. It's just that our body needs its time to make the adjustment according to the habit you changed.

3. You quit EVERYTHING at the same time. It is good to want to change your habits and it is good to want to be better than before. But it is also important not to strain your body all at once. Start by reducing carbohydrate intake slowly. Let 2 weeks pass and then reduce sugar. Let 2 weeks pass and then reduce bread or butter or oil or salt. What I want to say is that you have to make slow and steady steps. No major change took place overnight. Everything happened steadily and correctly. Make changes to your everyday life but with patience. What we want to achieve through this plan but also from every plan is to create a nice experience that will last more than the 3 months you need to achieve your specific goals. Create an experience and mentality of thinking that will hold on for the rest of your life.

4. The amount you use your screens over the course of the day. I do not propose to minimize its use in half or anything. I suggest that you do not use a monitor (mobile, tablet, or laptop) as soon as you wake up. Get up, drink coffee, eat breakfast or anything else you do in the morning and do not worry about screens for an hour. You will see that you wake up better and have better clarity about the goals of the day, but you are also more concentrated during the day. It is very important to give priority to yourself and not to the screen.

5. That you can have fun in whatever you do. This is also the basis for our third argument. What matters is to like what you do now and this trip you have started. Even a big part of it. So over 70% must please you. Do not do it until the 3 months have passed and then return to your old habits. It is important for us, as is for you, to do it and to continue on the same or similar way of life after that. What matters is to like what you are doing now and want to be better every day also after the end of the trainings. We want you to have a better lifestyle and after this training and nutrition cycle. What matters is to cultivate a better lifestyle in general. That's why we want you to make all that a part of your everyday life. Not just a piece of your life that has passed and gone. Experience this as much as you can and learn from each step and from each change. See how your body changes, but also the way you think about yourself and about your life in general. Do not let anything go unnoticed. Everything is done for some reason and you are currently changing for the best in your life. Learn to live with it and you will live your life better from now on. You deserve the best and you can get it one step at a time. Once you have finished this 3-month step, you will be able to carry on more actively and achieve any other goal. And go from good to great.

6. An hour after your workout it is very important to have a meal or take a supplement with protein and carbohydrates to replenish energy faster.

A good percentage for the post-training meal is as follows:

- Carbohydrates 50%
- Protein 30%
- Fat 20%

To achieve better protein synthesis, the meal should be at least one hour after training.

This meal is one of the most important because it helps us to repair the injured muscles during training and helps us to be stronger in the next few days in a similar or heavier training.

7. We don't recommend a protein shake right after your training cause you caused so much 'damage' on your muscles that your body needs about an hour to recover and get back to its regular rhythms. So if you drink a shake right after you will stall the protein synthesis and cause the opposite effect. The anabolic window as they say is 'open' 4-6 hours after your training. So your next 1 to 3 meals are as much important too.

And last but not least,

8. Training is when you have a goal to lose or gain weight. Training is organized. Has a beginning and an End. When you know what exercises you will be doing and why, you are going to train. When you go to the gym

without a goal, without knowing what you want to exercise, what the purpose of your workouts is and the only thing you do is exercise the mirror muscles (chest, arms, back) then you just workout. You don't train or do sports.

CHAPTER FOUR

BASIC METABOLIC RATE

INTRODUCTION TO YOUR DAILY AND TOTAL CALORIES

The total amount of energy (calories) needed by the body for all its vital functions in a resting state (contraction of the heart, breathing, hormone secretion, nervous system activity, etc.) is called ***Basic Metabolic Rate.***

Below is a table of decreasing or increasing daily calories that will help you a lot in your goals.

Body weight (kg) multiplied by A or B or C or D

A. 24,8	0-2 TRAININGS/WEEK
B. 26,4	1-3 TRAININGS/WEEK
C. 28,6	3-5 TRAININGS/WEEK
D. 30,8	6+ TRAININGS/WEEK

Result multiplied by 1 or 2 or 3 or 4

1. VERY LOW ACTIVITY:	1.1 minus 200
2. LOW ACTIVITY:	1.275 minus 300
3. MODERATE ACTIVITY:	1.350 minus 400
4. HIGH ACTIVITY:	1.750 minus 500

FOR A CALORIE SURPLUS:

In our total we add 200 or 300 calories if we have very low or low mobility accordingly.

Or add 400 or up to 550 calories if we have moderate or high mobility respectively.

We also round up the amount.

FOR A CALORIE DEFICIT:

Do as above but subtract the corresponding calories.

FOR MAINTENANCE:

We do the calculations, but we do not subtract or add calories to the total.

For example, for a 30-year-old man who weighs 56 kilos, has very low mobility and wants to gain weight then the equation is as follows:

$56 * 26.4 = 1478.4 * 1.1 = 1626.24 + 200 = 1826.24$. And with rounding we have 1850 or 1900 calories a day. That is, if he wants to gain weight in moderation. If you add 500 calories to this example probably you're going to end a fat trainee at the end of your workouts. Moderation is Key.

Do not forget that you have to walk at least 10,000 steps every day for the first 6 weeks and the next and final 6 weeks at least 15,000 steps. That way, you are always active. Also, at the weight loss stage you have to remember to do Cardio 4 to 5 times a week. Weight training burns fat because you train many muscle groups at once. You do 8 or 10 or 12 reps for 30 seconds and then rest for 30 to 45 seconds. That way you activate your body, then let it relax and then the same. So, your body uses both aerobic and anaerobic at the same time and you burn more fat.

And remember that what seems logical to you from outside the gym as to what to do to lose fat and to get muscle mass is exactly the opposite of what you have to do most of the times.

Our body operates very differently from our common sense.

Compound movements make our waist handle more weight in time so it also builds the strength of the abdomen.

So, if your goal is to lose or maintain weight you have to do the following:

Cardio 5%
HIIT 5%
Training with weights (Resistance training) 30%
Nutrition 60%

But if your goal is to gain weight, then you must do the following:

Cardio 1%
HIIT 2%
Training with weights (Resistance training) 47%
Nutrition 50%

TOTAL DAILY ENERGY EXPENDITURE

To calculate the details of your diet and your body rates, we must first make some calculations. Such as your total daily energy expenditure.

There is a great website where you can calculate it very quickly and know how many grams per macronutrients (protein, carbs, fat) you have to consume daily if you want to gain, lose or maintain your muscle mass!

Here is the site:

https://www.tdeecalculator.net

From here you can begin. It will ask you to put in your age, your weight, your height, your approximate fat percentage, and the number of trainings per week.

If this training program you will follow with us is your first and you hit the gym 2-3 times a week in average, then put in 3-5 times a week.

Then scroll down to "cutting" and take a look at the tabs. You will choose the one that says "low or moderate carb". With those percentages you can go to a dietician and give the exact information you want to get a diet that fits you exactly.

Below is my Sunday nutrition. The day I am off training I eat a little bit less or sometimes I fast for 20-24 hours. It's not much as far as cooking and preparation, because it contains fruit and nuts, cottage and some meals I can have with me in a lunch box at work.

BREAKFAST	100g MILK	100g CEREALS	
INTERMEDIATE	200g FRUITS	or Protein Shake	
NOON	120g Brown Rice	200gr. MEATBALL OR 200gr. FISH	HALF CUP COTTAGE CHEESE
TRAINING	WEIGHTS & CARDIO (45mins)	600-800kcal	
POST-TRAINING MEAL	200gr. FRUIT	or Protein Shake	
AFTERNOON	200gr. FRUIT W/ GREEK YOGURT		
DINNER 2	100g Brown Rice	200g MEATBALL OR 200g FISH	

Now let's just go over to the main issue, which is Macronutrients.

Total:

1. Carbohydrates – 290g
2. Protein - 130g
3. Fat - 32g
   Total calories = 2000 kcal

In general, try to note down the calories you consume every day in your meals.

You can get help on that from several apps on your smartphone where you can add whatever you eat or even scan the labels of the product and you get exactly the calories and the ingredients you consume.

Another option I would suggest, is to ask from your nutritionist a detailed day-by-day program according to the calories you wish to consume every day.

The solution to the problem is to take part in more than one solution.

Gymnastics, nutrition and aerobics and out-of-gym workout. With a single solution you never solve a problem caused by more problems in your life.

Accept your problem. You are who you are because of the choices you made.

Do not change what you are but the choices you make from now on. Your talents will not change. But your skills and knowledge will. Be yourself and you will fulfill more every day.

Challenge yourself

We include a section with challenges for your daily routine to empower you day by day and to make you believe in yourself even more. You can do it!!

CHALLENGE YOURSELF

15000 STEPS EVERY DAY	QUIT USING THE ELEVATOR FOR 2/3/4/5/6 WEEKS
PARK YOUR CAR FAR AWAY FROM WORK.	WALK YOUR BLOCK ONE OR TWO TIMES BEFORE YOU GET INSIDE YOUR CAR
WORK YOU CALVE MUSCLES AS YOU GO UP THE STAIRS	GET ONE STOP BACK FROM YOUR TERMINAL DESTINATION AND WALK
QUIT SUGAR FOR A WEEK OR TWO	QUIT WHITE BREAD AND COOKIES FOR A WEEK OR TWO
LIMIT ALCOHOL TO ONE DRINK PER WEEK AND/OR ONE DRINK PER TWO WEEKS	QUIT SODAS FOR ONE MONTH OR MORE
DON'T EAT BREAD WITH YOUR MEALS FOR A MONTH	READ A BOOK BEFORE YOU SLEEP
READ A BOOK BEFORE YOU LEAVE HOME	LISTEN TO SEMINARS AND AUDIOBOOKS DURING YOUR CARDIO
SPEND MORE TIME OUTSIDE	EAT OUT OR SWEETS ONLY ON SUNDAY
FAST FOR 20 HOURS THE DAYS YOU'RE NOT WORKING OUT. BEGIN THE PREVIOUS DAY	ONE DAY EAT ONLY FRUITS. EAT FRUITS DON'T DRINK JUICES

CHAPTER FIVE

INTRODUCTION TO STRETCHING DYNAMIC AND STATIC

Dynamic stretches are intended to warm up the muscles we are about to train to help our body respond better to the training. To avoid lack of range of motion and injuries during training.

Always remember to perform dynamic stretches before your trainings and at the end of them, do static stretches from 20'' to 30'' at each stretch for the exact same reason.

Stretches must be performed slowly and steadily to the point that we don't feel the muscle being stretched intensely. Otherwise, we get the opposite effect from stretching.

We provide you with pre-training (dynamic) and post-training stretches (static).

Let's begin!

DYNAMIC STRETCHING

UPPER BODY:

- Shoulder Rotations, 20 reps each
- Cable or Band External Rotation (back, rear delts) and Internal Rotation (chest, biceps)
- Scorpion mobility stretch
- Wall Slides
- Cat and Camel
- Rear belts w/ band

LOWER BODY:

- Squat with pause 20 seconds
- Split squat using bodyweight
- Leg swings (back and forth, right and left)
- Butterfly with movement
- RDL's with light weight
- Calves (standing and/or seated)

STATIC STRETCHING

UPPER BODY:

- Quadriceps from the standing position
- Adductor from the seated position
- Back femur from the standing position
- Gastrocnemius from the standing position
- Propionamide from the standing position
- Butterfly without movement

LOWER BODY:

- On the arm
- Forearm extension
- Side bending of the neck (left and right)
- Horizontal arm adduction
- Stretching the core on a horizontal bar
- Tricep extension behind the head (left and right arm)
- Bicep stretch (left and right)
- The child's pose
- Dog pose with down gradient on a wall
- Arms stretching in front of the chest with hands joined
- Arms stretching in our back with hands joined

CHAPTER SIX

THE FLIGHT OF ICARUS

The time we all have been waiting for has come. To make trainings a reality in order to prepare for the Flight of Icarus.

To be able to change yourself and your body for good and be able to Fly and Reach your Goals.

Now it's time to become stronger and see your body reach new levels of strength and hypertrophy. Start Icarus program and fear nothing.

Stay focused, strong and tuned in on our page at the end of this book.

Always remember:

Happiness is in the Process and not the Result

PREPPING PHASE

2 WEEKS OF STRENGTH TRAINING

These two weeks are a prepping phase for you. That means you are preparing to find out how many weights you can lift in order to know better yourself for the real workouts. Those workouts are going to help you get stronger so you can lift with proper and stronger form on the workouts that follow. An easy way to calculate your **1RM** is through this website:

https://exrx.net/Calculators/OneRepMax

So pay attention to your form. Perform the workouts slow and steady so you can understand every movement and set the basis of your workouts so you can strive on your Goals. Dont forget something really meaningful: You're doing this for Yourself. Have Fun And enjoy every Phase so it will last Longer in your life. Not only 12 Weeks.

Are you ready to get Shredded?

TRAINING INFO:
VOLUME 75% - 85% 1RM
REST: 180 seconds
FREQUENCY 5X/Week

Don't Forget:

10 MINUTES MOBILITY STRETCHING BEFORE TRAINING

AND 10 MINUTES STATIC STRETCHING AFTER TRAINING.

AND LOG YOUR WEIGHTS.

When you see a # it means you have to do a Drop Set on your last Set. Lower the weight 2 times in half.

DAY ONE: LEGS/ DELTS	SETS * REPS	WEIGHT / EXERCISE:
BACK SQUAT	5*5	
LEG PRESS	5*5	
LEG EXT.	5*6#	
STANDING CALVES	5*8#	
FRONT RAISES	5*10#	
CABLE CRUNCHES	4*12	

DAY TWO: PULL	SETS * REPS	WEIGHT / EXERCISE
RACK PULL	5*6	
PULL UPS (WEIGHTED)	5*6	
BENTOVER ROWS	5*8	
REAR-DELTS (cable)	4*10#	
BICEP CURLS (DB)	4*8	
INCLINE CURLS	4*10#	
WOOD CHOPS (high pulley)	4*12	

DAY THREE: LEGS/ DELTS	SETS * REPS	WEIGHT / EXERCISE
FRONT SQUATS	5*6	
SUMO DEADLIFTS	5*6	
LEG CURLS	5*8#	
CABLE PULL THROUGS	5*8	
MILITARY PRESS	5*6	
BICYCLE CRUNCHES	4*30	
STANDING CALVES	5*8#	

DAY FOUR: PUSH	SETS * REPS	WEIGHT / EXERCISE
CHEST PRESS	5*6	
DIPS	5*6	
CLOSE GRIP PRESS (BB)	5*8	
ROPE EXT.	5*8#	
SHOULDER PRESS	5*8	
PUSH PRESS	5*8#	
OTIS UPS (weighted)	4*12	

DAY FIVE: BACK/ CHEST	SETS * REPS	WEIGHT / EXERCISE
CHIN UPS	5*6	
DEADLIFTS	5*6	
CABLE ROWS	5*8	
INCLINE CHEST PRESS	5*8	
CHEST FLYS (DB)	5*8#	
PUSH UPS (AFAP)	5*FAIL	
PREACHER CURLS SS OVERHEAD EXT.	5*8#	
RUSSIAN TWISTS (weighted)	4*12	

PHASE ONE

HYPERTROPHY WEEKS 1 & 2 & 3

Those two weeks are hypertrophy based trainings. That means that you perform more repetitions (REPS) with more intensity.

We want the 10 REPS you perform to be your best reps and also be explosive. What you achieve is more endurance and also keeping your heartrate up.

That way you burn more calories and fat because you don't have much time to rest between sets. Between exercises you REST 45 to 60 seconds.

Those 3 weeks will make you feel more energized and give you more strength for the upcoming weeks.

Time to Push Yourself!

TRAINING INFO:

VOLUME 80% - 85% 1RM
REST 30" – 45"
FREQUENCY: 5x/Week

Don't Forget:

10 MINUTES MOBILITY STRETCHING BEFORE TRAINING
AND 10 MINUTES STATIC STRETCHING AFTER TRAINING.
AND LOG YOUR WEIGHTS.

When you see a # it means you have to do a Drop Set on your
last Set. Lower the weight 2 times in half.

DAY ONE: LEGS	SETS * REPS	WEIGHT / EXERCISE
BACK SQUATS	5*12,10,8,6,4	
WALKING LUNGES	4*10	
LEG EXT.	4*10#	
LEG PRESS CALVES	4*8*	
SINGLE LEG PRESS	4*10	
ADDUCTORS (machine)	4*10	
REAR DELTS (DB)	4*12*	
SHOULDER PRESS (DB-Unilateral)	4*12	
KNEELING WOOD CHOPS (low pulley) SS SUITCASE	3*12 SS 3*25 steps	

DAY TWO: PUSH	SETS * REPS	WEIGHT / EXERCISE
CHEST PRESS (DB)	5*12,10,8,6,4	
CROSSOVER (mid pulley)	4*10#	
DIPS SS PUSH UPS	4*10	
CABLE FLYS (low pulley)	4*10	
PECK DECK	4*10#	
ROPE EXT.	4*10	
REVERSE GRIP CURLS SS OVERHEAD EXT.	4*10	
KICKBACKS	4*10#	
HANGING LEG RAISES SS CABLE CRUNCHES	4*10	

DAY THREE: PULL	SETS * REPS	WEIGHT / EXERCISE
RACK PULLS	4*10	
PULL UPS	4*FAIL	
DUMBBELL ROWS VS PULLDOWNS	4*10	
T-BAR	4*10#	
SINGLE STRAIGHT ARM PULLDOWNS	4*10	
INCLINE CURLS	4*10	
BICEP CURLS	4*10#	
WRIST CURLS	4*10	
PLANK	4*60sec	

DAY FOUR: LEGS	SETS * REPS	WEIGHT / EXERCISE
RDL'S	5*12,10,8,6,4	
HIP THRUST	4*10	
SINGLE LEG CURLS	4*10	
LEG PRESS (upper stance)	4*10#	
STANDING CALVES	4*10*	
CABLE PULL THROUGHS	4*10	
FRONT RAISES	4*10#	
UPRIGHT ROWS SS SHOULDER PRESS (BB)	4*10	
ACCORDION CRUNCHES WEIGHTED SS ACCORDION BODYWEIGHT	4*12	

DAY FIVE: PUSH/PULL	SETS * REPS	WEIGHT / EXERCISE
INCLINE PRESS	5*12,10,8,6,4	
CABLE FLYS (high pulley)	4*10#	
LANDMINE PRESS	4*10	
INCLINE PRESS (DB-lower angle than 45°)	4*10#	
SINGLE ARM ROWS	4*10	
SHRUGS SS LATERAL RAISES	4*10	
REAR DELTS SS INVERTED ROWS	4*10	
HAMMER CURLS SS BARBELL CURLS	4*10	
BACK EXTENSIONS	4*10	

PHASE TWO

STRENGTH WEEKS 4 & 5

Those two weeks are high volume in order for your muscles to grow stronger as you perform those workouts. What you have to do is to perform them slow and steady when the weights are heavier.

Don't you ever forget how important are the Strength Weeks for your overall muscle endurance and your Hypertrophy.

Those two weeks are hybrid performed. Which means we have low reps (4-6 and high reps (8 -15) Reps. Rest Time between exercises is 90 seconds.

It's your time to become Stronger!

TRAINING INFO:

VOLUME 80% - 90% 1RM

REST 70"-90"

FREQUENCY: 5x/Week

Don't Forget:

10 MINUTES MOBILITY STRETCHING BEFORE TRAINING
AND 10 MINUTES STATIC STRETCHING AFTER TRAINING.
AND LOG YOUR WEIGHTS.

DAY ONE: BACK/ DELTS	SETS * REPS	WEIGHT / EXERCISE
RACK PULLS	5*6,6,4,4,4	
CABLE ROWS	4*8	
LAT PULLDOWNS	5*6,6,4,4,4	
STRAIGHT ARM PULLDOWNS	4*8	
FRONT RAISES (cable)	4*8	
REAR DELTS	4*8	
CHIN DOWNS	4*8	
CABLE CRUNCHES SS FLATTER KIKCS	4*15	

DAY TWO: PUSH	SETS * REPS	WEIGHT / EXERCISE
CHEST PRESS (BB)	5*6,6,4,4,4	
DIPS (weighted)	5*6,6,4,4,4	
INCLINE PRESS	5*6,6,4,4,4	
CLOSE GRIP PRESS	5*6,6,4,4,4	
OVERHEAD EXT. (unilateral)	4*8	
SKULL CRUSHER	4*8	
LEG RAISES SS ACCORDION CRUNCHES (weighted)	4*15	

DAY THREE: LEGS	SETS * REPS	WEIGHT / EXERCISE
BACK SQUAT	5*6,6,4,4,4	
WALKING LUNGES	4*8	
FRONT SQUATS	5*6,6,4,4,4	
SINGLE LEG EXT.	4*12	
SIDE LEG KICKS	3*15	
SEATED CALVES	4*15	
RUSSIAN TWISTS SS BICYCLE CRUNCHES	4*15	

DAY FOUR: ARMS	SETS * REPS	WEIGHT / EXERCISE
PUSH PRESS	5*6,6,4,4,4	
INCLINE FRONT RAISES	4*8	
REAR DELTS (cable)	4*8	
FACE PULLS	4*8	
CONCENTRATED CURLS (cable)	4*8	
LATERAL RAISES (cable)	4*10	
BARBELL CURLS	4*8	
SIDE PLANK	4*20sec	

DAY FIVE: LOWER	SETS * REPS	WEIGHT / EXERCISE
HIP THRUSTS	5*6,6,4,4,4	
RDL'S	4*8	
SINGLE LEG CURLS	4*8	
SEATED CALVES	4*15	
LEG PRESS (feet up and sumo)	4*8	
LYING HAM CURLS	4*10	
JUMP SQUATS	4*10	
KNEELING WOOD CHOPS	4*15	

PHASE THREE

We are back on track with the Hypertrophy protocol. Those three weeks are going to be tough. And when we say tough we mean STRONG AS HELL.

It's almost over because we're on the middle of the workouts but when you finish week number 6 you wish it was really over. Those weeks are going to make you fitter than ever and get you closer to your goals.

They're going to be hard but you're going to be stronger and faster. Rest Time Between Exercises is going to be 45 seconds for those workouts.

Be Prepared to Conquer Yourself!

TRAINING INFO:

VOLUME: 75% 1RM

REST: 25"-40"

FREQUENCY: 6x/Week

Don't Forget:

10 MINUTES MOBILITY STRETCHING BEFORE TRAINING
AND 10 MINUTES STATIC STRETCHING AFTER TRAINING.
AND LOG YOUR WEIGHTS.

When you see a # it means you have to do a Drop Set on your
last Set. Lower the weight 2 times in half.

DAY ONE: PUSH	SETS * REPS	WEIGHT / EXERCISE
MILITARY PRESS	5*5	
BENCH PRESS (BB) SS CLOSE GRIP PRESS (DB)	4*10	
CHEST PRESS (DB-lower angle than 45°)	5*10#	
CABLE FLYS (high pulley) SS PUSH UPS	5*10	
PECK DECK	5*10#	
LYING TRICEP EXT	5*10	
ROPE EXT.	5*10#	
LEG RAISES SS MOUNTAIN CLIMBERS	4*10 SS 20	

DAY TWO: PULL	SETS * REPS	WEIGHT / EXERCISE
DEADLIFTS	5*5	
T-BAR ROWS SS REAR DELTS (DB)	5*10	
SHOULDER Y-LIFTS (cable)	5*10#	
LAT PULLDOWNS SS STRAIGHT ARM PULLDOWNS	5*10	
BENTOVER ROWS	5*10	
REVERSE CURLS SS PREACHER CURLS (ez bar)	5*10	
UNILATERAL BICEP CURLS	5*10#	
WEIGHTED CRUNCHES SS PLANK	4*10 SS 30sec	

DAY THREE: LEGS	SETS * REPS	WEIGHT / EXERCISE
BACK SQUATS	5*5	
LEG PRESS (stiff legs) SS JUMP SQUAT (BW)	5*10 SS 10	
LEG EXT.	5*10#	
SPRINT	5*30sec	
SEATED CALVES	5*15#	
BOX SIDE STEP UPS	5*10	
QUAD ISO HOLD (weighted)	5*25sec#	
BACK EXTENSIONS	4*12	

DAY FOUR: PUSH	SETS * REPS	WEIGHT / EXERCISE
KICK BACKS	5*10	
SKULL CRUSHERS	5*10	
OVERHEAD EXT.	5*10#	
LANDMINE PRESS	5*10#	
DUMBBELL FLYS	5*10#	
TRICEPS DIPS	5*10	
ARNOLD PRESS	5*10	
SUITCASE	3*25steps	
SIDE PLANK	3*30sec	

DAY FIVE: PULL	SETS * REPS	WEIGHT / EXERCISE
CHIN DOWS	5*5	
LATERAL RAISES VS FRONT RAISES	4*10	
REVERSE STRAIGHT ARM PULLDOWNS	5*10#	
SHRUGS	5*10#	
FACE PULLS	5*10	
INCLINE DUMBBELL CURLS	5*10	
BICEP CURLS (cable)	5*10	
ACCORDION CRUNCHES SS CABLE CRUNCHES	5*12,12,12,15,15	

DAY SIX: LEGS	SETS * REPS	WEIGHT / EXERCISE
RDL'S	5*5	
SINGLE LEG CURLS	5*10	
DONKEY KICKS (cable)	5*10	
CABLE PULL THROUGHS	5*10#	
SEATED CALVES	5*10	
SIDE KICKS (cable)	5*10	
HIP THRUSTS (DB)	5*12#	
REAR DELTS (machine)	5*10#	
SIDE PLANK CRUNCHES	5*12,15,12,15,12	

PHASE FOUR

DELOAD WEEK 9

So, we're glad you make it so far and we're celebrating this event by offering you a DELOAD WEEK. Its that week when you perform in less intensity in order for your muscles to rest after all that stress you've caused on them.

This way your body is going to reward you by showing you all the muscles that grow all that time. You'll see your body pumped more than before. That's the result of letting your body rest. It rewards you with the aesthetics of your workouts.

Do your trainings, but, everyday for 5 days do 30 minutes Cardio of light Jogging. That means jogging to the point you can breath normal. Not the other way. Enjoy this week and don't feel guilty of not working out so intensively!

Relax Physically and Mentally!
TRAINING INFO:

VOLUME 70%± 1RM

REST 60"-90"

FREQUENCY: 4x/Week

Don't Forget:

10 MINUTES MOBILITY STRETCHING BEFORE TRAINING
AND 10 MINUTES STATIC STRETCHING AFTER TRAINING.
AND LOG YOUR WEIGHTS.

DAY ONE: PULL	SETS * REPS	WEIGHT / EXERCISE
RACK PULLS	3*12	
PULL DOWNS	3*12	
CABLE ROWS	3*12	
BARBELL CURLS	3*12	
HAMMER CURLS	3*12	
WOOD CHOPS (low pulley)	3*12	

DAY TWO: PUSH	SETS * REPS	WEIGHT / EXERCISE
BENCH PRESS	3*12	
PECK DECK	3*12	
FLYS (DB-flat)	3*12	
ROPE EXT.	3*12	
CLOSE GRIP PRESS (DB)	3*12	
RUSSIAN TWISTS	3*12	

DAY THREE: LEGS / DELTS	SETS * REPS	WEIGHT / EXERCISE
FRONT SQUAT	3*12	
LEG CURLS	3*12	
GLUTE BRIDGE	3*12	
STANDING CALVES	3*12	
REAR DELTS (DB)	3*12	
CABLE CRUNCHES	3*20	

DAY FOUR: UPPER/ LOWER	SETS * REPS	WEIGHT / EXERCISE
BENTOVER ROWS	3*12	
SHRUGS	3*12	
FLOOR PRESS	3*12	
CABLE PULL THROUGHS	3*12	
LEG EXT.	3*12	
BACK EXT. (BW)	3*12	

PHASE FIVE

So it's the last Phase of the Icarus Workouts. Its going to be extremely hard and painful, but you have to fly over to your Goals. It's the Last 3 weeks and you're going to be the best. The last week (No.12) rest between exercises 1 minute and not only 20 seconds. This way you'll progress more!

Don't you ever forget why you started and who you want to become. Don't just do the workouts and Game Over. Do all that for a long time. Like forever. Have fun and enjoy every process of your life.

You're going to change for the better and you have to do it everyday. Be yourself and discover yourself through a more fit way!

Time to Rock those Workouts!

TRAINING INFO:

VOLUME 80% - 90% 1RM
REST 15" – 25"
FREQUENCY: 6x/Week

Don't Forget:

10 MINUTES DYNAMIC STRETCHES BEFORE TRAINING
AND 10 MINUTES STATIC AFTER TRAINING.
AND LOG YOUR WEIGHTS.

When you see a # it means you have to do a Drop Set on your
last Set. Lower the weight 2 times in half.

DAY ONE: PUSH	SETS * REPS	WEIGHT / EXERCISE
CHEST PRESS (BB)	6*8	
FLYS (DB-flat)	6*8#	
CROSSOVER (high pulley)	6*8#	
DIPS	6*8	
PECK DECK	6*8	
KICK BACKS	6*8#	
FRENCH PRESS (cable)	4*20	
LEG RAISES	6*15	

DAY TWO: PULL	SETS * REPS	WEIGHT / EXERCISE
CABLE V-ROWS	6*8	
REAR DELTS	6*8#	
BENTOVER ROWS	6*8	
BARBELL SHRUGS	6*8#	
STRAIGHT ARMS PULLDOWNS	6*8#	
BICEP CURLS	6*8#	
HAMMER CURLS	6*8	
PULLOVER	6*8	
CABLE CRUNCHES	6*15	

DAY THREE: LEGS	SETS * REPS	WEIGHT / EXERCISE
FRONT SQUATS	6*8	
LEG PRESS (low feet and narrow)	6*8#	
GOBLET SQUAT AND PAUSE	6*8	
UNILATERAL SEATED CALVES	6*15	
LEG EXT.	6*8#	
SHOULDER PRESS (DB)	6*8#	
FRONT RAISES	6*10	
SINGLE LEG EXT.	5*10#	
SIDE PLANK	4*45sec	

DAY FOUR: PUSH	SETS * REPS	WEIGHT / EXERCISE
PUSH PRESS	6*8	
CLOSE GRIP PRESS	6*8#	
ROPE EXT.	6*8#	
FRENCH PRESS (chin)	6*8	
OVERHEAD EXT (CABLE)	6*8	
INCLINE FLYS	6*8#	
PECK DECK	6*8#	
INCLINE FLYS	6*8#	
BENCH TRICEPS DIPS	6*10#	
PLANK	4*60sec	

DAY FIVE: PULL	SETS * REPS	WEIGHT / EXERCISE
INCLINE BICEP CURLS	6*8#	
E-Z BAR REVERSE CURLS	6*8	
E-Z BAR PREACHER CURLS	6*8#	
SPIDER CURLS	6*10	
V-GRIP PULLDOWNS	6*8#	
ROWS (machine)	6*8	
LATERAL RAISES	6*8#	
UPRIGHT ROWS	6*10#	
HANGING LEG RAISES SS BICYCLE CRUNCHES	4*15	

DAY SIX: LEGS	SETS * REPS	WEIGHT / EXERCISE
HIP THRUSTS & 5sec PAUSE (DB)	6*10	
SUMO SQUATS & PAUSE 3sec (DB)	6*10	
PULL THROUGHS	6*8#	
LEG CURLS	6*8	
SEATED CALVES	6*14#	
CURTSY LUNGES or SIDE KICKS	6*10	
JUMP SQUATS (weighted)	6*10	
RDL'S	6*8	
BACK EXT.	4*10	

CONGRATULATIONS!

YOU DID IT!

You've just finished THE FLIGHT OF ICARUS WORKOUTS. Now you are ready to challenge yourself more and acquire more than you have previously thought possible!

You have come to a good muscular level and now it's time to think if you want to do another round of Cutting training or if you want to do a round to maintain the weight you gained and the fat you've lost.

The decision is yours. Whatever it is, share your experience with us and leave a comment on our page on Instagram and also on Amazon for us to find out what you think of our program for cutting and losing fat.

Check also our last book about Hypertrophy

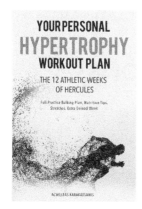

Your Personal Hypertrophy Workout Plan

THE 12 ATHLETIC WEEKS OF HERCULES

Full Practice Bulking Plan, Nutrition Tips, Stretches, Extra Deload Week

The ultimate goal about gaining muscle mass (bulking) can be on your hands with 12 weeks training, Nutrition Tips, Macros and supplements analysis, Extra Deload Week and an example of our meals to get ahead with your goals and make a Clean Bulk.

Gaining muscle is difficult because except the hard work on the gym you have to work hard on the kitchen. It's a tricky phase because everyone thinks its only reckless eating all the time-pizza, tacos, burgers, donuts, waffles and the list goes on and on. But that's not the case. The real case is a hard workout and a flexible nutrition to keep you going.

With that in mind check our Book about Hypertrophy Training and get ahead of others trying to Bulk up fast eating all the wrong meals and training hearing bro-science and ending in Snap-City with all the other guys and girls!

Make yourself a favor and get well prepared with our 12 Athletic Weeks of Hercules!

ABOUT THE AUTHOR

ACHILLEAS KARAKATSANIS is a certified personal trainer who loves fitness and a healthy nutrition lifestyle.

He lives in Athens and Santorini, Greece. Achilleas loves writing and reading books, watching and creating videos and inspiring his trainees to build their physique and a strong Mindset.

Make sure to watch our training videos in our page on Instagram:

https://www.instagram.com/aka_achilles/

Check our last Book in Amazon:

and feel free to contact us on:

achilleas.ebooks@hotmail.com

Made in the USA
Monee, IL
13 October 2022